YOUR KNOWLEDGE HAS VALUE

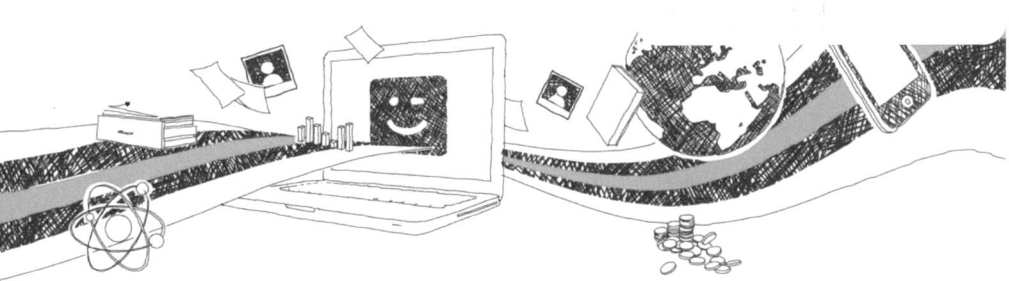

- We will publish your bachelor's and master's thesis, essays and papers

- Your own eBook and book - sold worldwide in all relevant shops

- Earn money with each sale

Upload your text at www.GRIN.com and publish for free

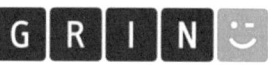

Bibliographic information published by the German National Library:

The German National Library lists this publication in the National Bibliography; detailed bibliographic data are available on the Internet at http://dnb.dnb.de .

This book is copyright material and must not be copied, reproduced, transferred, distributed, leased, licensed or publicly performed or used in any way except as specifically permitted in writing by the publishers, as allowed under the terms and conditions under which it was purchased or as strictly permitted by applicable copyright law. Any unauthorized distribution or use of this text may be a direct infringement of the author s and publisher s rights and those responsible may be liable in law accordingly.

Imprint:

Copyright © 2017 GRIN Verlag, Open Publishing GmbH
Print and binding: Books on Demand GmbH, Norderstedt Germany
ISBN: 9783668581944

This book at GRIN:

http://www.grin.com/en/e-book/382797/reducing-maternal-mortality-in-liberia-by-increasing-the-information-dissemination

Baba Sillah

Reducing Maternal Mortality in Liberia by Increasing the Information Dissemination for Maternal Education

GRIN Publishing

GRIN - Your knowledge has value

Since its foundation in 1998, GRIN has specialized in publishing academic texts by students, college teachers and other academics as e-book and printed book. The website www.grin.com is an ideal platform for presenting term papers, final papers, scientific essays, dissertations and specialist books.

Visit us on the internet:

http://www.grin.com/

http://www.facebook.com/grincom

http://www.twitter.com/grin_com

Increasing Information Dissemination for Maternal Education: A Strategy for Reducing Maternal Mortality in Liberia

Baba Sillah
MA Student, Graduate School of Global Studies, Sophia Jochi University, Tokyo, Japan.

Abstract

This paper argues that the lack of a continuous, serious and robust government-driven and coordinated information dissemination program in Liberia on the importance of antenatal care among a highly illiterate population constitutes significant impediment to the overall goal to reducing maternal mortality and contributes to the high rate of maternal mortality. The argument is founded on two fundamental observations. These observations include: the high illiteracy rate in Liberia and its contribution to maternal mortality and, the underutilization improved and expanded maternal health facilities and services. We see these two points as mutually reinforcing and that one will not fare well in the absence of the other. We conclude with five precursory recommendations and emphasize that if any policy to reduce maternal mortality in Liberia is to be successful, holding all other factors constant, such policy must include a deliberate program for increasing information dissemination for maternal education.

Keywords: Maternal mortality, information dissemination, antenatal care, illiteracy, Liberia healthcare

Table of Contents

Introduction 3
An Overview of Maternal Mortality 3
A Review of Liberia's very high Maternal Mortality 4
A case for improving information dissemination for combating maternal mortality 5
   1. The high illiteracy rate in Liberia and its contribution to high maternal mortality 6
   2. The underutilization of relatively improved and expanded maternal health facilities and services 8
Discussion 9
Findings, conclusion and recommendations 10
Bibliography 11

Introduction

This topic is significant for some fundamental reasons. First, it reviews the current high maternal mortality trend in Liberia and its causes as well as where the health sector places emphasis in its efforts to reverse the troubling trend. Second, given that the government of Liberia does not have any continuous, serious and robust information dissemination program, as we could not find such in the policy documents reviewed, this paper argues that not much consideration is being given to the potential that increasing information dissemination has for enhancing maternal education and thereby contributing to a decrease in the current high maternal mortality rate in Liberia. The paper posits that illiteracy is a major factor in the high maternal mortality rate in Liberia. In support of this postulate we look at relevant data on literacy from Liberia and found high levels of illiteracy especially among women. Third, the paper looks at the level of improvements in the health sector of the country particularly; regarding maternal care and argues that, though it still leaves much to be desired, if pregnant women are regularly provided with the necessary information regarding the importance of maternal care, doctor's visit, where to seek maternal care and how often to do so, this will promote the education and change of attitude the combination of which will influence them to utilize existing maternal health services more and to take other proactive health measures.

This paper argues that given the high illiteracy rate in Liberia notwithstanding the improvements in health delivery care, the reasons behind the high increase in maternal mortality may not be fully accounted for only by low emergency obstetrics, high home deliveries by unskilled personnel and shortage of midwives. That level of education, it has been shown, has significant function in whether a country does well in its maternal mortality ratings or not.

Therefore this paper attempts to make a case that while efforts are being made to further improve emergency obstetrics; reduce home deliveries by unskilled personnel and shortage of midwives, among others, all of which are indispensable to a properly functioning maternal health system, the lack of information dissemination on the importance of antenatal care among a highly illiterate population constitutes significant impediment to the overall goal of reducing maternal mortality and contributes to the high rate of maternal mortality.

An Overview of Maternal Mortality

Maternal mortality is defined as the death of a pregnant woman during pregnancy, or within 42 days of termination of pregnancy, regardless of the duration and the site of the pregnancy, as long as the death is due to cause (s) connected to or exacerbated by the pregnancy or its management. This includes direct or indirect obstetric death and excludes accidental or incidental causes.[1] Every day, approximately 830 women die from preventable causes related to pregnancy and childbirth, 99% of all such deaths happen in developing countries.[2] Maternal mortality is higher in women living in rural areas and among poorer communities. Young adolescents face a higher risk of complications and death as a result of pregnancy than other women.[3] While it still high as it is currently, it is im-

---

[1] International Classification of Diseases (ICD), International Classification of Diseases, Volume-2 Instruction Manual.10th Revision, Geneva, World Health Organization, 2010). ((Accessed July 12, 2017).)
[2] World Health Organization, Maternal Mortality, Fact Sheet 2016 (Accessed July 14, 2017)
[3] Maternal-perinatal morbidity and mortality associated with adolescent pregnancy in Latin America: Cross-sectional study. Conde-Agudelo A, Belizan JM, Lammers C. American Journal of Obstetrics and Gynecology,2004, 192:342–349

portant to note that between 1990 to 2015 maternal mortality worldwide dropped by about 44%. The Sustainable Development Goals successor program to the Millennium Development Goals seeks to reduce maternal mortality to 70 deaths per 100, 000 live births globally between 2016 and 2030.[4] Women in developing countries on average, have many more pregnancies than women in developed countries. This situation makes their lifetime risk of death due to pregnancy higher. The probability that a 15-year old woman will eventually perish due to maternal causes is 1 in every 4,900 persons in developed. In countries designated as fragile states, the risk is 1 in 54; showing the consequences from breakdowns in health systems.[5]

The phenomenon of maternal mortality remains very high in sub-Saharan Africa though progress against it is being achieved in all regions of the world. The good news is that, since most maternal deaths result from preventable causes, almost all maternal deaths can be prevented. There is no gainsaying that poverty contributes to maternal mortality. According to the UNICEF, this is evidenced by the huge disparities found between the richest and poorest countries. Additionally, the risk of maternal death in high-income countries is 1 in 3,300 contrasted with 1 in 41 in low-income countries.[6]

A Review of Liberia's very high Maternal Mortality

Liberia currently has one of the highest burdens of maternal mortality in the world.[7] The Ministry of Health of Liberia attributes this to low emergency obstetrics, high home deliveries by unskilled personnel and shortage of midwives.[8] The trend has been steadily deteriorating from 578 per 100, 000 live births in 2005[9] to 990 per 100,000 live births in 2011.[10] Currently maternal mortality in Liberia is approximated to stand at around 1,072 per 100,000 live births as of 2015.[11] This makes Liberia one of the countries with the highest maternal mortality rates in the world.[12] According to the UNICEF Liberia 2012-2017 country programme document, the trend has worsened in spite of improvement in antenatal care.[13]

What is most troubling is that the entire increasing trend in maternal mortality is happening amidst significant improvements in the Liberian health sector. The World Health Organization in its Country Cooperation Strategy of 2017 reports an increase by 27% in the functional health facilities of the country between 2010 and 2016. The same report also indicates important upturns in key interventions areas including antenatal coverage and immunization. The report also mentions a decline from 41% in 2008 to 29% in 2015 of the population that has to travel more than 1 hour to access health facility. Additionally, the reports shows that the per capita expenditure on healthy has increased

---

[4] SDG Goal-3
[5] World Health Organization, Maternal Mortality, Fact Sheet 2016 (Accessed July 14, 2017)
[6] UNICEF Data: Monitoring the Situation of Children and Women
[7] 8Ministry of Liberia of Liberia, Investment Case for Reproductive, Maternal New Born, Child, and Adolescent Health 2016-2020
[8] Ibid.
[9] Liberia Demographic Health Survey (LDHS 2000).
[10] Human Development Report (2011).
[11] Liberia Demographic Health Survey (LDHS 2013).
[12] World Bank.Maternal mortality ratio (modeled estimate, per 100 000 live births).((Accessed July 12, 2017).)http://data.worldbank.org/indicator/SH.STA.MMRT?locations=LR
[13] UNICEF Liberia country programme document 2012-2017 ((Accessed July, 12 2017).)

from less than US$20 to 21% in 2000 to US$46 in 2014 and that out-of-pocket expenditure accounted for 21% of total health expenditure.[14]

In its September 2015 report to the UN Secretary-General, Mr. Bin Ki-Moon, the Government of Liberia reaffirmed its commitment to the Global Strategy for Women's and Children' Health launched in 2010, and outlined some gains as well as challenges including the Ebola onslaught in 2014 to achieving some key milestones. However, the government did not make any specific mention of the need or importance of information dissemination as an element of its sustainable action to end maternal mortality.

Unfortunately, through all of the policy documents and reports we accessed for this paper, there was not seen any nationwide, aggressive government-coordinated information dissemination program to educate women and men on the danger of maternal mortality and what actions to take to prevent it.

A case for improving information dissemination for combating maternal mortality

While the relatively weak presence and poor quality of healthcare may seem the putative reason for this for high maternal mortality in Liberia, these alone may not give a fuller understanding of the phenomenon. The thinking that availability, accessibility, and affordability of healthcare facilities are the sole factors for determining maternal health care or health in general is problematized by the fact that human behavior and choices play important roles in decision making.[15] We believe that the lack of proper information to pregnant women on how and where to seek prenatal care, and to encourage them to do so is a key factor that may explain the high maternal mortality level in Liberia.

Data from Demographic Health Surveys in Liberia indicate low utilization of basic healthcare particularly in rural areas where only 25.5 percent of women delivered by health professionals.[16] These factors combined, controlling for others, including shortage of midwives and other economic problems, are important for reinforcing the perspective that the high maternal mortality burden of Liberia may be due to the fact that pregnant women are not fully utilizing the available health services because of the lack of information which could influence their behavior to increase doctor's visit and utilize existing services more.

Interestingly, in all the policy documents reviewed including the SDG Goal-3 on Strategy for Women's, Children and Adolescents' Health, the Indicator and Monitoring Framework for the Global Strategy on the Strategy for Women's, Children and Adolescents' Health (2016-2030) of the Health Ministry of Liberia of Liberia, Investment Case for Reproductive, Maternal New Born, Child, and Adolescent Health 2016-2020, Liberia Demographic Health Survey (LDHS 2013, UNICEF Liberia country programme document 2012-2017, no case was made for aggressive government-driven information dissemination on maternal mortality. Even though much emphasis is

---

[14] Country Cooperation Strategy of 2017
[15] Phillips KA, Morrison KR, Andersen R, Aday LA, Health Serv Res. 1998 Aug; 33(3 Pt 1):571-96.
(Accessed July, 122017).)
[16] Kruk ME, Rockers PC, Varpilah ST, Macauley R. Which doctor?: Determinants of utilization of formal and informal health care in post-conflict Liberia. Med Care. 2011;49(6):585–591. doi:
10.1097/MLR.0b013e31820f0dd4.[PubMedCrossRef(Accessed July 12, 2017).)

placed on strengthening health systems, ensuring universal health coverage for comprehensive reproductive, maternal, and newborn care, among others, no particular attention is given to the importance of information dissemination as a tool for providing maternal education to pregnant women and which will influence them to access existing services more and as a way of preventing mortality and decreasing overall death rates.

Thus this paper argues that massive government coordinated information dissemination to promote education on antenatal care and the importance of doctor's visit will contribute to decreasing maternal mortality. The argument is founded on two fundamental observations. These observations include (1) the high illiteracy rate in Liberia and its contribution to maternal mortality (2); the underutilization improved and expanded maternal health facilities and services. We see these two points as mutually reinforcing and that one will not fare well in the absence of the other.

1. The high illiteracy rate in Liberia and its contribution to high maternal mortality

As of 2015, the literacy rate based on demographics of Liberians age 15 and above stood at 62.4% for males and 32.8% for females. Liberia has one of the highest illiteracy rates in the world and ranks 189 on the Index Mundi demographic literacy chart with an overall illiteracy rate of 60.8%. The Liberia Demographic and Health Survey (LDHS) of 2007 indicate 17% of women ages 45—49 years are literate, compared with 62% of men. Although the discrepancies in literacy by sex have declined among the younger generations, large gaps remain: only 58% of women age 15—19 years are literate, compared with 73% of men age 15—19 years.[17] Though comparison of data from the 2013 LDHS with the 2007 LDHS shows some improvement in educational attainment among women, the proportion of women attaining literary education is still very disproportionate to that of men. The LDHS 2013 indicate that, between 2007 and 2013 the proportion of those ages 15-19 that completed primary school increased from 31 to 41 percent for females and from 36 to 46 percent for males. Among those ages 20-24, the proportions that completed primary school increased from 40 to 53 percent among women and from 64 to 76 percent among men.[18] The above statistics on education in Liberia point to the fact that illiteracy is higher among women and may be one of the key underpinning factors contributing to the country's high maternal mortality.

As education serves as a vital element for informed decision making, pregnant women who are illiterate may not understand the full importance of maternal care and the significance of doctor's visit and as a result risk losing their lives before taking the necessary precautions to prevent death. Education helps people build the kind of behaviors and habits that are beneficial to good health. Studies have shown strong correlation between maternal education and decrease in maternal level of mortality. For example, according the University of North Carolina at Chapel Hill School of Medicine published in the Science Daily in May 2012, a scientific analysis of 50 years of maternal mortality data from Chile led by Dr. Elard Koch, an epidemiologist and author of the study, found that the most important factor for reducing maternal mortality is the education of women. Among other things, the publication quotes Koch as saying: "In fact, during 2008, the overall MMR declined again, to 16.5 per 100,000 live births, positioning Chile as the country with the second lowest ratio

---

[17] Africa Health Observatory, World Health Organization Regional Office for Africa (Accessed July, 12 2017).)
[18] Liberia Demographic and Health Survey (2013:23) (Accessed July, 12 2017).

in the American continent after Canada and with at least two points lower MMR than United States."

The study also proved that apart from other contributing variables to this decrease including predictable factors of delivery by skilled health workers, complimentary nutrition for pregnant women, etc, the most significant factor and the one which buoyed the effectiveness of the others was the educational level of women. In fact, every additional year of maternal education there was a corresponding decrease in maternal mortality rate of 29.3 per 100, 000 births. Additionally the study confirmed that apart from other contributing variables to this decrease including predictable factors of delivery by skilled health workers, complimentary nutrition for pregnant women, etc, the most significant factor and the one which buoyed the effectiveness of the others was the educational level of women. In fact, with every additional year of maternal education there was a corresponding decrease in maternal mortality rate of 29.3 per 100, 000 births.[19]

Illiterate women are unable and less likely to take the personal initiative to read up on critical steps they must take to avoid complications during pregnancy and maternal mortality. One obvious challenge which could discourage them from undertaking such personal initiative is the inability to read. This strengthens the case that when women in Liberia who are pregnant and of childbearing age are provided maternal education through deliberately designed and coordinated government publicity program on what measures they must take to prevent maternal mortality, there is much plausibility that the current troubling percentage of maternal mortality in the country will be reduced. While publicity is not meant to substitute for academic literary education, it can be use as an immediate and medium term measure to provide essential information while the country works on improving formal education. The Liberia Core Welfare Indicator Survey (CWIQ) of 2007 showed that contraceptive prevalence rate (CPR) is 7.7% among women with secondary education in Liberia and 20.6% among women without secondary education.[20] At the time, only 1.1% of rural women had completed secondary school (LDHS 2007). This makes for a strong correlation between the illiteracy rate in the country and the high maternal mortality rate.

A project for the reduction of maternal morbidity and mortality in Liberia under the United Nations Trust Fund for Human Security, implemented by the United Nations Family Planning Association (UNFPA) and the World Health Organization between May 2008 and December 2009 had as one of its objectives, the promotion of knowledge on sexual and reproductive health among vulnerable groups including adolescents. The direct beneficiaries of the project were 301,040 women of childbearing age resident in the following counties Bomi, Nimba, Bong, Grand Bassa, Maryland, Grand Gedeh and Rivercess. At the end of the project, one of the notable achievements was the improvement of the quality of maternal health services through the expansion of the knowledge of existing maternal health providers, knowledge of the number of skilled attendants, including the availability of appropriate instruments. It was highlighted that the project also focused on training traditional midwives (TTM) on how to educate pregnant women on how to identify complication

---

[19] Elard Koch, John Thorp, Miguel Bravo, Sebastian Gatica, Camila X. Romeo, Heman Aguilera, IyonneAhlers. Women's Education Level, Maternal Health Facilities, Abortion Legislation and Maternal Deaths: A Natural Experiment in Chile from 1957 to 2007. (Accessed July 12, 2017).
[20] Liberia Core Welfare Indicator Survey (2007).

and risks to maternal morbidity and mortality.[21] That the above project which key objective was to reduce maternal morbidity and mortality placed emphasis on expanding knowledge of the existing maternal health providers, knowledge of available attendants and training traditional midwives to educate pregnant women on how to identify complications and take actions to prevent maternal mortality, says a lot about the significance of information dissemination for reducing maternal mortality in Liberia especially in rural areas of the country.

2. The underutilization of relatively improved and expanded maternal health facilities and services

According to the World Health Organization African Health Observatory, infrastructure includes buildings, their plant and equipment; utilities such as power and water supply; waste management; and transport and communication. It also involves investment decisions, with issues of specification, price and procurement and considering the implications of investment in facilities, transport or technologies for recurrent costs, staffing levels, skill needs and maintenance systems (http://www.aho.afro.who.int/profiles_information/index.php/Liberia:Service_delivery_-_The_Health_System). Liberia's almost two-decade long civil war had devastating effects on it health infrastructure. The conflict also left in its wake a huge demand for qualified health practitioners. At the end of the conflict in 2003 only 51% of the health amenities were operational as a result it was approximated that only 10 % of the overall population could access basic health services. In responding to the dire situation with the health system, the Liberia government instituted the Basic Package of Health Services BPHS, a range of evidenced-based, cost-effective interventions to improve the population health. Services in high demand were identified and prioritized across the health sector. However by 2010 80% of government clinics were estimated to meet minimum standards for delivery of BPHS and therefore the government scaled up the BPHS to Essential Package of Health Services EPHS by 2011.[22]

Improvements have been made in reducing the distance that women once had to travel to seek maternal care. From a survey conducted in Konobo district in South Eastern Liberia, seventy-three percent of women (CI 60-84%) had to travel for more than two hours in and before 2007 to access the nearest clinic. This figure experienced dramatic reduction with only 32% of women in 2013 reporting same.[23] The challenges in the health sector are nothing near being fully addressed, howbeit, some progress is has been made in improving infrastructure and personnel. While the health system is still saddled with personnel, equipment and infrastructure challenges, the Ministry of Health and Social Welfare report of 2011, points out that Ninety-six percent of women age 15-49 who had a live birth in the five years preceding the survey received prenatal care from a skilled provider (doctor, nurse, midwife, or physician's assistant) during their last pregnancy. This figure represents

---

[21] UN Trust Fund for Human Security, Reduction of Maternal Morbidity and Mortality in Liberia December (2009)

[22] Liberia Ministry of Health and Social Welfare, Essential Package of Health Services, Monrovia, Liberia: 2011. Available online at: http://apps.who.int/medicinedocs/documents/s198008en.pdf. (Accessed July 23, 2017).

[23] Katherine Kentoffio, John D. Kraemer, Rajesh Panjabi, et al, G. Andrew Sechler, Stephen Selinsky and Mark "Charting health system reconstruction in post-war Liberia: a comparison of rural vs.remote healthcare utilization." BMC Health Services Research, 2016. http://creativecommons.org/publicdomain/zero/1.0

a significant departure from what was reported in the Liberia Demographic Health Survey LDHS of 2007.

Additionally, eighteen percent of women received care from a doctor, 76 percent from a nurse or midwife, and 2 percent from a physician's assistant. Only 2 percent of women received care from a traditional midwife or other unskilled provider, as compared with 17 percent of women in the 2007 LDHS. Two percent of women received no prenatal care, as compared with 4 percent in the 2007 LDHS.
The Ministry of Health and Social Welfare of Liberia credits these improvements in the provision of prenatal care by skilled providers to the increased number of, and geographic access to, health facilities and increased numbers of skilled providers across Liberia in recent years (MOHSW, 2011).

Health accreditation which is recommended by the WHO to African countries as a way of formulating national health quality provision programmes has also informed Liberia's knowledge about the current capacity of its health sector. The country lacked accreditation process in the past as a result the Ministry of Health and Social Welfare did not have a clear database on the number, location and qualifications of government-employed health care workers and healthcare facilities. The accreditation process brought to light additional information, identifying 437 open health facilities in late 2008, of which 349 are government-owned. As of 2009, more than 70% of the government health facilities are operated on behalf of the MOHSW by faith-based organizations or 1 of 15 international and local NGOs. This information is important because, it helps the case that though still inadequate, it is not the lack of health personnel, equipment and facilities that may be solely responsible for high rate of maternal mortality as the lack of adequate information on the importance of antenatal care and where to find it is also critical to consider.

Discussion

As the above information reveals, the trend in maternal mortality has been steadily deteriorating from 578 per 100, 000 live births in 2005 to 990 per 100,000 live births in 2011. Currently maternal mortality in Liberia is approximated at that around 1,072 per 100,000 live births as of 2015. However, all the policy health policy documents and reports on Liberia as reviewed on for this paper did not have any deliberate, robust government coordinated and executed information dissemination program with the objective of providing maternal education to pregnant women or women in general regarding the importance of maternal care especially antenatal care, as well as where to seek care and whom to seek care from. We also did not find any clear policy about getting information to pregnant women about the kinds of services that are available and how they can access them. The Ministry of Health and Social Welfare though constrained by budgetary inadequacies is also more focused on low emergency obstetrics, high home deliveries by unskilled personnel and shortage of midwives, and health infrastructure. While the MoHW's focus is not misdirected, designing and rolling out programs that will educate and inspire trust in women to utilize the facilities and personnel already available. It is worth noting, however, that the impact that increasing the information dissemination and utilization of existing maternal health facilities will have on maternal mortality in

Liberia can only be fully understood when current maternal mortality data are compared to data on maternal mortality in a post-information dissemination environment.

Findings, conclusion and recommendations

Based on the high figures of illiteracy among women, this paper finds that maternal mortality is high in Liberia due to high illiteracy rate among women which is contributing to the low utilization of existing qualified health personnel and facilities. Additionally this paper finds that the Ministry of Health of Liberia does not have a deliberate, continuous, serious and robust government-driven and coordinated information dissemination program to educate women on the importance of antenatal care. This paper affirms as other researchers have also, that education helps people build the kind of behaviors and habits that are beneficial to good health.

Studies have shown strong correlation between maternal education and decrease in maternal level of mortality. Thus the Ministry of Health of Liberia is encouraged to take some proactive actions, working with partners in the development and health community to reach women and inform them about the importance of maternal health, where to seek it, whom to seek it from and how often to seek it. It is important to note that in this paper we have controlled for economic and financial factors because we believe that a woman with money but without the appropriate information is just as vulnerable to maternal mortality as a woman without money and without education. Information dissemination will stir a move toward enhancing hospital visits, reducing risky behaviors during pregnancy, gaining awareness of proper nutrition and food, increasing hospital deliveries and ultimately reducing maternal mortality rate.

Finally, this paper states that if any policy to reduce maternal mortality in Liberia is to be successful, holding all other factors constant, such policy must include a deliberate program for increasing information dissemination for maternal education. The following recommendation covering policy and practical measures though not exhaustive are here provided for consideration:

1. That the Ministry of Health and Social Welfare establish an Anti-Maternal Mortality information secretariat (AMMIS).

2. That the Anti-maternal mortality information secretariat designs a comprehensive anti-Maternal Mortality information dissemination program.

3. That the Anti-maternal mortality information secretariat will train specified community elderly women to discuss the importance of maternal health with pregnant women. This should be done at the community or neighborhood level.

4. That a maternal health information dissemination center is established in each county with a mandate to plan and execute quarterly maternal health information.

5. That the Ministry of Health and Social Welfare encourage a change in attitude among women and encourage them to utilize services of trained midwives and access health facilities often.

Bibliography

Katherine Kentoffio, John D. Kraemer, Thomas Griffiths, Avi Kenny, Rajesh Panjabi, G. Andrew Sechler, Stephen Selinsky and Mark J. Siedner, "Charting health system reconstruction in post-war Liberia: a comparison of rural vs.remote healthcare utilization." BMC Health Services Research, 2016. http://creativecommons.org/publicdomain/zero/1.0

Maternal-perinatal morbidity and mortality associated with adolescent pregnancy in Latin America: Cross-sectional study.Conde-Agudelo A, Belizan JM, Lammers C. American Journal of Obstetrics and Gynecology, 2004, 192:342–349.

Government of Liberia: OFM Extract for MOHSW Annual Report. 2010, Monrovia: Ministry of Health & Social Welfare

Government of Liberia: Ministry of Health & Social Welfare: 2009 BPHS Accreditation: Final Results Report. 2009, Monrovia: Ministry of Health & Social Welfare

Varpilah et al; Rebuilding human resources for health: a case study from Liberia; Licensee BioMed Central Ltd. 2011

Liberia Institute of Statistics and Geo-Information Services, Ministry of Health and Social Welfare, National AIDS Control Program, and Macro International Inc. 2008

World Bank.Maternal mortality ratio (modeled estimate, per 100 000 live births).((Accessed July 12, 2017).)http://data.worldbank.org/indicator/SH.STA.MMRT?locations=LR

Cleveland, E. C., Dahn, B. T., Lincoln, T. M., Safer, M., Podesta, M., & Bradley, E. (2011). Introducing health facility accreditation in Liberia. Global Public Health, 6(3), 271–282. http://doi.org/10.1080/17441692.2010.489052 (Accessed July 25, 2017

Country Cooperation Strategy of 2017

SDG Goal-3 on Strategy for Women's, Children and Adolescents' Health

Essential Package of Health Services EPHS by (2011), Ministry of Health and Social Welfare of Liberia

YOUR KNOWLEDGE HAS VALUE

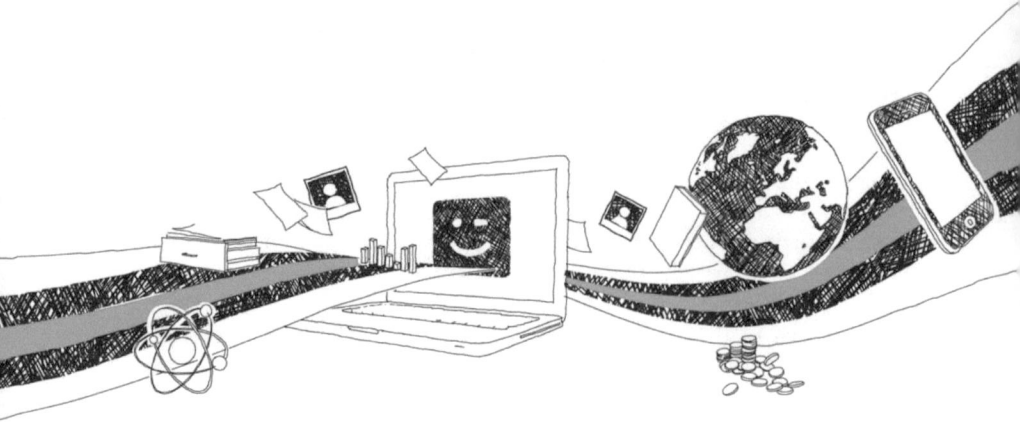

- We will publish your bachelor's and
  master's thesis, essays and papers

- Your own eBook and book -
  sold worldwide in all relevant shops

- Earn money with each sale

Upload your text at www.GRIN.com
and publish for free

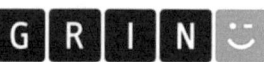